More From Love's
Little Instruction Book

More From Love's
Little Instruction Book

Romantic Hints for Lovers of All Ages

Annie Pigeon

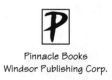

Pinnacle Books
Windsor Publishing Corp.

PINNACLE BOOKS are published by

Windsor Publishing Corp.
850 Third Ave
New York, NY 10022

The P logo Reg. U.S. Pat. & TM off. Pinnacle is a trademark of Windsor Publishing Corp.

First Printing: February, 1995

Printed in the United States of America

For Clark Kent

1. Tell him you had a sexy dream about him.

♥

2. Build her a roaring campfire.

♥

3. Have a midlife crisis together.

♥

4. See how your last names would sound hyphenated.

♥

5. Save for retirement together.

♥

6. At bed and breakfasts, skip the breakfast.

♥

7. Tell her you loved her in a past life, too.

♥

8. Take her to a movie with no chase scene.

♥

9. Never say, "You look tired."

♥

10. Never say, "You're aging well."

♥

11. Play "What will we name our kids?"

♥

12. Play "What will they name our grandkids?"

♥

13. Meditate together.

♥

14. Remember, your parents are just as weird as his parents.

♥

15. Pour a head on his beer.

♥

16. Teach the kids to say, "Mommy's pretty."

♥

17. Teach your parrot to say it, too.

♥

18. Don't needle.

♥

19. Don't wheedle.

♥

20. Persist, but don't insist.

♥

21. Never put her on hold.

♥

22. Sew his shirt button back on.

♥

23. Call when you get there so he doesn't worry.

♥

24. On a scale of one to ten, tell her she's an eleven.

♥

25. Tell her she's getting "too thin."

♥

26. Post a "Top Ten Reasons I Love You" list on the fridge.

♥

27. Enter a talent show together.

♥

28. Retype his résumé.

♥

29. Don't correct his grammar in public.

♥

30. Tell her "You look even prettier without make-up."

♥

31. Tell her you'd rather cuddle than watch the game.

♥

32. Let him watch the game.

♥

33. Don't mention her soufflé has fallen.

♥

34. Write his name in the sand.

♥

35. Write her name in skywriting.

♥

36. Carve your initials in wood.

♥

37. Take a hayride.

♥

38. Take a sleighride.

♥

39. Ride a cable car.

♥

40. Give her a locket.

♥

41. Have his boss to dinner.

♥

42. Climb to the top of the lighthouse.

43. Take a long walk in the woods.

♥

44. Send her on a shopping spree.

♥

45. Learn how to buy a diamond.

♥

46. Whatever he says, look impressed.

♥

47. Whatever she says, look interested.

♥

48. Never issue an ultimatum.

♥

49. Tell him your sun sign goes well with his moon.

♥

50. Tell her her aura's aglow.

♥

51. Break the routine.

52. Change the toilet paper roll yourself.

53. Find her lost contact lens.

54. Get her sweater when it's chilly.

55. Get his slippers when he's lazy.

56. Be the one to bring in the paper when it's raining.

♥

57. Mail a letter for her.

♥

58. Return his library book.

♥

59. Take some things at face value.

♥

60. Don't ask, "Do you talk to your shrink about me?"

♥

61. Don't ask, "Does your mother really like me?"

♥

62. Tell him he looks great in Bermuda shorts.

♥

63. Never tease her for ordering dessert.

♥

64. Don't snoop.

♥

65. Don't sneak.

♥

66. Don't listen in on the extension.

♥

67. Okay, not everyone looks great in Spandex.

♥

68. Okay, not everyone looks great in thong bikinis.

♥

69. Never say, "Isn't that outfit a little young for you?"

♥

70. Buy matching terrycloth robes.

♥

71. Stroke her knee.

♥

72. Stroke his ego.

♥

73. Play footsie under the dinner table.

♥

74. Build something together.

♥

75. Pack him a gourmet lunch.

♥

76. Pump air in her bicycle tires.

♥

77. Frame her favorite photograph.

♥

78. Alphabetize his record collection.

♥

79. Help him clean his closets.

♥

80. Run her bath.

♥

81. Pull over when you spot wildflowers.

♥

82. Give yourselves a party.

♥

83. Carry hankies scented with each other's
perfume or cologne.

♥

84. Entice.

♥

85. Be nice.

♥

86. Make a little sacrifice.

♥

87. Remember that no relationship's paradise.

♥

88. Do a mating dance.

♥

89. Let him browse *Sports Illustrated*'s swimsuit edition.

♥

90. Have lunch on a terrace.

♥

91. Garden together.

♥

92. Remember, sharing colds and flus is still sharing.

♥

93. Send the kids to Grandma's.

♥

94. Make a daisy chain.

♥

95. Recycle together.

♥

96. Sponsor an endangered species together.

♥

97. Don't spend too much time debating health care reform.

98. Republicans and Democrats can so co-exist.

99. Send a love note on E-mail.

100. Ring his modem.

101. Don't mess with his software.

102. Don't crash her hard drive.

♥

103. Don't crash his Harley.

♥

104. Make home-made ice cream.

♥

105. Learn to square dance.

♥

106. Serenade her.

♥

107. Take a mud bath together.

♥

108. Loofah her.

♥

109. Give him a pedicure.

♥

110. Try aromatherapy together.

♥

111. Tell her she doesn't need liposuction.

♥

112. Drink something sparkling.

♥

113. (No Cold Duck, please.)

♥

114. Bake her homemade bread.

♥

115. Watch his yeast rise.

♥

116. Go with him to the auto show.

♥

117. Go with her to the health spa.

♥

118. No heckling while she exercises.

♥

119. Have her portrait painted.

♥

120. Make him homemade pasta.

♥

121. Take a hot tub together.

♥

122. Share some sushi.

♥

123. Visit his Aunt Elsie in the nursing home.

♥

124. A steam iron is not a gift.

♥

125. A weed-eater is not a gift.

♥

126. Pick apples together.

♥

127. Make jam together.

♥

128. Learn to windsurf together.

♥

129. Tour a winery.

♥

130. Ride a merry-go-round.

♥

131. Read her palm and praise her love line.

♥

132. Read his Tarot cards and praise his spread.

♥

133. Get out the old lava lamp.

♥

134. Try a ouija board together.

♥

135. Rent *The Piano*.

♥

136. *Don't rent Indecent Proposal*.

♥

137. Share an oversized umbrella.

♥

138. Sing in the rain.

♥

139. Whistle in the dark.

♥

140. Have a snowball fight.

♥

141. Take in a fireworks display.

♥

142. Forgive the bad.

♥

143. Relive the good.

♥

144. Waltz.

♥

145. Laugh at his schmaltz.

♥

146. Do the limbo.

♥

147. Do the mambo.

♥

148. Share a comfortable silence.

♥

149. Tour Tuscany.

♥

150. Tour Burgundy.

♥

151. Tour the neighborhoods where you grew up.

♥

152. Write living wills.

♥

153. Don't show each other up.

♥

154. Don't have showdowns.

♥

155. Feed the ducks.

♥

156. Surprise her with a call from an airplane.

♥

157. Get up early with the kids so she can sleep late.

♥

158. Make him some cappucino.

♥

159. Eat a mango together.

♥

160. Let her raid your closet.

♥

161. Trim the wedding budget and spend it on the honeymoon.

♥

162. Hold hands while you snorkle.

♥

163. Write your names in cake icing.

♥

164. Write them on each other's body.

♥

165. Flatter.

♥

166. Chatter.

♥

167. Share a small bed.

♥

168. Be a little possessive.

♥

169. If she doesn't like it, don't do it.

♥

170. If you know he likes it, do it a lot.

♥

171. Understand if he has to be out of town.

♥

172. Get her her own toolbox.

♥

173. Add her name to your lease.

♥

174. Spring for the orchestra seats.

♥

175. Tell him he inspires you.

♥

176. Tell her she's your muse.

♥

177. Say, "Those laugh lines become you."

♥

178. Tell him how funny he is.

♥

179. Say, "I owe it all to you."

♥

180. Book the honeymoon suite just for fun.

♥

181. So she had a little fender bender.

♥

182. Order her second-choice entrée and give her a bite.

♥

183. Make her name a tattoo.

♥

184. Neatness counts.

♥

185. Table manners couldn't hurt.

♥

186. Blush.

♥

187. Don't rush.

♥

188. Surprise him by doing his chore once in a while.

♥

189. Let him be cranky while he quits smoking.

♥

190. Let her be cranky while she's on a diet.

191. Learn to cook his family's favorite dish.

♥

192. Never take each other for granted.

♥

193. Share paying the bills.

♥

194. Don't laugh when she shrieks at a bug.

♥

195. Admire her gluteal muscles.

♥

196. Play "your" song on the jukebox.

♥

197. Get up early when he has to.

♥

198. Don't put skim milk in his coffee.

♥

199. Don't put real sugar in her tea.

♥

200. Be outrageous.

♥

201. Take Italian lessons together.

♥

202. Recreate the first meal you ever shared.

♥

203. Revisit the place where you met.

♥

204. Give her a charm bracelet.

♥

205. Look for rainbows together.

♥

206. Find four-leaf clovers together.

♥

207. Stay out of each other's family feuds.

♥

208. Say it with roses.

♥

209. Say it with pearls.

♥

210. Say it with chocolate truffles.

♥

211. Above all, just say it.

♥

212. Plan a fantasy vacation together.

♥

213. Refill his mug.

♥

214. Sit in his lap.

♥

215. Give her cat a cuddle.

♥

216. Give his dog a bone.

♥

217. Paint her toenails.

♥

218. Braid her hair.

♥

219. Play Ginger Rogers and Fred Astaire.

♥

220. Never ask, "Didn't you used to be taller?"

♥

221. Say, "Someday our dentures will spend the night side by side."

♥

222. Let her drive once in a while.

♥

223. Assure her she's prettier than her passport photo.

♥

224. Amble.

♥

225. Window shop.

♥

226. Do nothing together.

♥

227. Tell her she's got shapely ankles.

♥

228. Teach him to use the Cuisinart.

♥

229. Teach her to use a wrench.

♥

230. Fix him a midnight snack.

♥

231. If she hates the goatee, shave it off.

♥

232. If he hates platinum blond, go back to natural.

♥

233. On your anniversary, send a thank-you note to whoever introduced you.

♥

234. Come up with code words for "I love you" to say in public.

♥

235. Give each other some elbow room.

♥

236. Don't open a restaurant together.

♥

237. Love does so mean having to say you're sorry.

♥

238. Say, "You must have been a beautiful baby."

♥

239. Say, "I hope our kids look just like you."

♥

240. Let him use your good guest towels.

♥

241. Pack him a thermos full of something hot.

♥

242. If you like different salad dressings, buy both.

243. Help her reach something high up.

♥

244. Help her buy a used car.

♥

245. Help him buy curtains.

♥

246. In winter, go south together at least once.

♥

247. Put your own dishes in the dishwasher.

♥

248. Spray Miracle-Gro on her potted plants.

♥

249. Don't ask, "Do you ever fantasize about anyone else?"

♥

250. Don't ask him to suck in his gut.

♥

251. Don't offer to buy her a girdle.

♥

252. Don't offer to buy him a toupée.

♥

253. Let her dad tell you war stories.

♥

254. Let his mom tell you childbirth stories.

♥

255. Remember his folks' anniversary.

256. Rub cocoa butter on her pregnant tummy.

♥

257. Tell her she has a beautiful soul.

♥

258. Promise to slow dance only with each other.

♥

259. Serve his chili extra hot.

♥

260. Tantrums happen.

♥

261. Oversights happen.

♥

262. Grouchiness happens.

♥

263. Shortcomings are endearing.

♥

264. Perfection is boring.

♥

265. Tell her you'd marry her all over again.

♥

266. Let him win at gin rummy.

♥

267. Make him a banana split.

♥

268. Buy her a rocking chair.

♥

269. Buy him a fountain pen.

♥

270. Let him rent the jet skis.

♥

271. Let him go to baseball camp.

♥

272. Take a steambath together.

♥

273. Serve him veggies you grew yourself.

274. Buy him a *Calvin and Hobbes* collection.

♥

275. Ask to see her old Barbie dolls.

♥

276. Ask to see his old baseball cards.

♥

277. Don't dish her friends.

♥

278. Give her something with her birthstone in it.

♥

279. Take a third honeymoon.

♥

280. Join a picket line together.

♥

281. Paint a picket fence together.

♥

282. Renew your wedding vows.

♥

283. If you get her answering machine, don't hang up.

♥

284. Call her your beauty queen.

♥

285. Call him your Romeo.

♥

286. Never be rude.

287. Don't cop an attitude.

288. No "I told you so's", please.

289. If a psychic says you'll leave him, leave the psychic.

290. Play Scarlett to his Rhett.

♥

291. Play Bogart to her Bacall.

♥

292. Write to say, "Miss you."

♥

293. Call just to say hi.

♥

294. Hail a cab for her.

♥

295. Rub his temples when he's tense.

♥

296. Swoon a little.

♥

297. Bat your eyes.

♥

298. Order one ice cream soda, two straws.

♥

299. Sit on a porch swing.

♥

300. Ride a paddle boat across a lake.

♥

301. Tell him he smells great.

♥

302. Remind her to slow down.

♥

303. Remind him to calm down.

♥

304. Offer to slay a dragon for her.

♥

305. Hug her after a nightmare.

♥

306. Work up a sweat together.

♥

307. Squeeze her fresh orange juice.

♥

308. Pop him some popcorn.

♥

309. Watch your wedding video.

♥

310. Tell him you wished you'd known him when he was a boy.

♥

311. Tell her you wish you'd taken her to her prom.

♥

312. Take a snow day together.

♥

313. Fall asleep with your head on his shoulder.

♥

314. Throw another log on the fire.

♥

315. Keep dinner warm when she's working late.

♥

316. Make sure his socks match.

♥

317. Start a tradition.

♥

318. Scribble your names in cement.

♥

319. Try a new cuisine together.

♥

320. Play a duet.

♥

321. Play fair.

♥

322. Fight fair.

♥

323. Let him be the first to flip through the paper.

♥

324. Don't open her magazines if she hasn't.

♥

325. Let her pick the mutual fund.

♥

326. Don't spy on his old girlfriends.

♥

327. Offer to burn your little black book.

♥

328. Try to learn something about his favorite sport.

♥

329. Schmooze each other's parents.

♥

330. Volunteer for a cause she cares about.

♥

331. Humor him.

♥

332. Praise her fashion sense.

♥

333. Know when to refrain from comment.

♥

334. Offer her the seat with the view.

335. Surprise her with a limo ride.

336. Tell a pregnant wife she's never looked better.

337. Don't make light of her soap opera.

338. Don't make her pump her own gas.

339. Share your frequent-flyer miles.

♥

340. Don't leave the mess for someone else to clean up.

♥

341. Don't leave the towels on the floor.

♥

342. Let him stretch the truth once in a while.

♥

343. Write a love song for her.

♥

344. Be tolerant.

♥

345. Don't antagonize.

♥

346. Don't agonize, either.

♥

347. Welcome him home with a surprise.

♥

348. Do your best.

♥

349. Don't be a pest.

♥

350. Once in a while, experiment.

♥

351. Watch your language.

♥

352. Watch the late show with her when she can't sleep.

♥

353. Take a night course together.

♥

354. Hold on tight in a thunderstorm.

♥

355. Ride an overnight train in a sleeper car.

♥

356. Go leaf-peeping each autumn.

♥

357. Call up her mother on Mother's Day.

♥

358. Have a shirt custom made for him.

♥

359. Buy her a politically correct fake fur.

♥

360. Switch movie seats when someone tall sits in front of her.

♥

361. Start planning for New Year's Eve 2000.

♥

362. Wish each other good luck.

♥

363. Say a prayer for each other.

♥

364. Pledge to reincarnate together.

♥

365. Stop and think what your life would be without each other.